# EPIDEMIOLOGY FOR THE UNINITIATED

## Fourth edition

# EPIDEMIOLOGY FOR THE UNINITIATED

## Fourth edition

### D COGGON, PHD, DM, FRCP, FFOM

*Reader in Occupational and Environmental Medicine,
Medical Research Council Environmental Epidemiology Unit,
University of Southampton, Southampton General Hospital,
Southampton*

### GEOFFREY ROSE, DM, DSC, FRCP, FFPHM

*late Emeritus Professor of Epidemiology, Department of Epidemiology,
London School of Hygiene and Tropical Medicine, London*

### D J P BARKER, PHD, MD, FRCP, FFPHM, FRCOG

*Professor of Clinical Epidemiology and Director,
Medical Research Council Environmental Epidemiology Unit,
University of Southampton, Southampton General Hospital,
Southampton*

BMJ
Publishing
Group

12378

WA
105
COC

First published 1979
Third impression 1983
Second edition 1986
Second impression 1987
Third impression 1989
Fourth impression 1990
Fifth impression 1992
Third edition 1993
Fourth edition 1997
Second impression 1999
Third impression 2000

**British Library Cataloguing in Publication Data**

A catalogue record for this book is available from the British Library.

ISBN 0-7279-1102-3

Typeset and printed by Latimer Trend & Company Ltd, Plymouth

# Contents

# 1: What is epidemiology?

Epidemiology is the study of how often diseases occur in different groups of people and why. Epidemiological information is used to plan and evaluate strategies to prevent illness and as a guide to the management of patients in whom disease has already developed.

Like the clinical findings and pathology, the epidemiology of a disease is an integral part of its basic description. The subject has its special techniques of data collection and interpretation, and its necessary jargon for technical terms. This short book aims to provide an ABC of the epidemiological approach, its terminology, and its methods. Our only assumption will be that readers already believe that epidemiological questions are worth answering. This introduction will indicate some of the distinctive characteristics of the epidemiological approach.

## All findings must relate to a defined population

A key feature of epidemiology is the measurement of disease outcomes in relation to a *population at risk*. The population at risk is the group of people, healthy or sick, who would be counted as cases if they had the disease being studied. For example, if a general practitioner were measuring how often patients consult him about deafness, the population at risk would comprise those people on his list (and perhaps also of his partners) who might see him about a hearing problem if they had one. Patients who, though still on the list, had moved to another area would not consult that doctor. They would therefore not belong to the population at risk.

The importance of considering the population at risk is illustrated by two examples. In a study of accidents to patients in

1

hospital it was noted that the largest number occurred among the elderly, and from this the authors concluded that "patients aged 60 and over are more prone to accidents." Another study, based on a survey of hang gliding accidents, recommended that flying should be banned between 11 am and 3 pm, because this was the time when 73% of the accidents occurred. Each of these studies based conclusions on the same logical error, namely, the *floating numerator*: the number of cases was not related to the appropriate "at risk" population. Had this been done, the conclusions might have been different. Differing *numbers* of accidents to patients and to hang gliders must reflect, at least in part, differing numbers at risk. Epidemiological conclusions (on risk) cannot be drawn from purely clinical data (on the number of sick people seen).

Implicit in any epidemiological investigation is the notion of a *target population* about which conclusions are to be drawn. Occasionally measurements can be made on the full target population. In a study to evaluate the effectiveness of dust control measures in British coal mines, information was available on all incident (new) cases of coal workers' pneumoconiosis throughout the country.

More often observations can only be made on a *study sample*, which is selected in some way from the target population. For example, a gastroenterologist wishing to draw general inferences about long term prognosis in patients with Crohn's disease might extrapolate from the experience of cases encountered in his own clinical practice. The confidence that can be placed in conclusions drawn from samples depends in part on sample size. Small samples can be unrepresentative just by chance, and the scope for chance errors can be quantified statistically. More problematic are the errors that arise from the method by which the sample is chosen. A gastroenterologist who has a special interest in Crohn's disease may be referred patients whose cases are unusual or difficult, the clinical course and complications of which are atypical of the disease more generally. Such systematic errors cannot usually be measured, and assessment therefore becomes a matter for subjective judgement.

Systematic sampling errors can be avoided by use of a random selection process in which each member of the target population has a known (non-zero) probability of being included in the study sample. However, this requires an enumeration or *census* of all members of the target population, which may not be feasible.

Often the selection of a study sample is partially random. Within the target population an accessible subset, the *study population*, is defined. The study sample is then chosen at random from the study population. Thus the people examined are at two removes from the group with which the study is ultimately concerned:

*Target population→study population→study sample*

This approach is appropriate where a suitable study population can be identified but is larger than the investigation requires. For example, in a survey of back pain and its possible causes, the target population was all potential back pain sufferers. The study population was defined as all people aged 20–59 from eight communities, and a sample of subjects was then randomly selected for investigation from within this study population. With this design, inference from the study sample to the study population is free from systematic sampling error, but further extrapolation to the target population remains a matter of judgement.

The definition of a study population begins with some characteristic which all its members have in common. This may be *geographical* ("all UK residents in 1985" or "all residents in a specified health district"); *occupational* ("all employees of a factory," "children attending a certain primary school", "all welders in England and Wales"); *based on special care* ("patients on a GP's list", "residents in an old people's home"); or *diagnostic* ("all people in Southampton who first had an epileptic fit during 1990–91"). Within this broad definition appropriate restrictions may be specified—for example in age range or sex.

## Oriented to groups rather than individuals

Clinical observations determine decisions about individuals. Epidemiological observations may also guide decisions about individuals, but they relate primarily to groups of people. This fundamental difference in the purpose of measurements implies different demands on the quality of data. An inquiry into the validity of death certificates as an indicator of the frequency of oesophageal cancer produced the results shown in table I.

Inaccuracy was alarming at the level of individual patients. Nevertheless, the false positive results balanced the false negatives so the clinicians' total $(53 + 21 = 74$ cases) was about the same as the pathologists' total $(53 + 22 = 75$ cases). Hence, in this instance, mortality statistics in the population seemed to be about right,

TABLE I—*Cause of death diagnosed clinically compared with at necropsy*

| Diagnosis of oesophageal cancer | No |
|---|---|
| Diagnosed by clinician and confirmed by pathologist | 53 |
| Diagnosed by clinician but not confirmed by pathologist | 21 |
| First diagnosed post mortem | 22 |

despite the unreliability of individual death certificates. Conversely, it may not be too serious clinically if Dr X systematically records blood pressure 10 mm Hg higher than his colleagues, because his management policy is (one hopes) adjusted accordingly. But choosing Dr X as an observer in a population study of the frequency of hypertension would be unfortunate.

## Conclusions are based on comparisons

Clues to *aetiology* come from comparing disease rates in groups with differing levels of exposure—for example, the incidence of congenital defects before and after a rubella epidemic or the rate of mesothelioma in people with or without exposure to asbestos. Clues will be missed, or false clues created, if comparisons are biased by unequal ascertainment of cases or exposure levels. Of course, if everyone is equally exposed there will not be any clues—epidemiology thrives on heterogeneity. If everyone smoked 20 cigarettes a day the link with lung cancer would have been undetectable. Lung cancer might then have been considered a "genetic disease", because its distribution depended on susceptibility to the effects of smoking.

Identifying *high risk* and *priority groups* also rests on unbiased comparison of rates. The *Decennial Occupational Supplement of the Registrar General of England and Wales* (1970–2) suggested major differences between occupations in the proportion of men surviving to age 65:

TABLE II—*Men surviving to 65, by occupation*

| | |
|---|---|
| Farmers (self employed) | 82% |
| Professionals | 77% |
| Skilled manual workers | 69% |
| Labourers | 63% |
| Armed forces | 42% |

These differences look important and challenging. However, one must consider how far the comparison may have been distorted either by inaccurate ascertainment of the deaths or the populations at risk or by selective influences on recruitment or retirement (especially important in the case of the armed forces).

Another task of epidemiology is *monitoring* or *surveillance* of time trends to show which diseases are increasing or decreasing in incidence and which are changing in their distribution. This information is needed to identify emerging problems and also to assess the effectiveness of measures to control old problems. Unfortunately, standards of diagnosis and data recording may change, and conclusions from time trends call for particular wariness.

The data from which epidemiology seeks to draw conclusions are nearly always collected by more than one person, often from different countries. Rigorous *standardisation* and *quality control* of investigative methods are essential in epidemiology; and if an apparent difference in disease rates has emerged, the first question is always "Might the comparison be biased?"

# 2: Quantifying disease in populations

## What is a case?

Measuring disease frequency in populations requires the stipulation of diagnostic criteria. In clinical practice the definition of "a case" generally assumes that, for any disease, people are divided into two discrete classes—the affected and the non-affected. This assumption works well enough in the hospital ward, and at one time it was also thought to be appropriate for populations. Cholera, for instance, was identified only by an attack of profuse watery diarrhoea, which was often fatal; but we now know that infection may be subclinical or cause only mild diarrhoea. Similarly for non-infectious diseases today we recognise the diagnostic importance of premalignant dysplasias, in situ carcinoma, mild hypertension, and presymptomatic airways obstruction. Increasingly it appears that disease in populations exists as a continuum of severity rather than as an all or none phenomenon. The rare exceptions are mainly genetic disorders with high penetrance, like achondroplasia; for most acquired diseases the real question in population studies is not "Has the person got it?" but "How much of it has he or she got?"

One approach, therefore, is to use measures that take into account the quantitative nature of disease. For example, the distribution of blood pressures in a population can be summarised by its mean and standard deviation. For practical reasons, however, it is often helpful to dichotomise the diagnostic continuum into "cases" and "non-cases". In defining the cut off point for such a division, four options may be considered:

*Statistical*—"Normal" may be defined as being within two standard deviations of the age specific mean, as in conventional laboratory practice. This is acceptable as a simple guide to the limits of what is common, but it must not be given any other importance because it fixes the frequency of "abnormal" values of every variable at around 5% in every population. More importantly, what is usual is not necessarily good.

*Clinical*—Clinical importance may be defined by the level of a variable above which symptoms and complications become more frequent. Thus, in a study of hip osteoarthritis cases were defined as subjects with a joint space of less than 2 mm on $x$ ray, as this level of narrowing was associated with a clear increase in symptoms.

*Prognostic*—Some clinical findings such as high systolic blood pressure or poor glucose tolerance may be symptomless and yet carry an adverse prognosis. Sometimes, as with glucose tolerance, there is a threshold value below which level and prognosis are unrelated. "Prognostically abnormal" is then definable by this level.

*Operational*—For some disorders, none of the above approaches is satisfactory. In men of 50, a systolic pressure of 150 mm Hg is common (that is, "statistically normal"), and it is clinically normal in the sense of being without symptoms. It carries an adverse prognosis, with a risk of fatal heart attack about twice that of a low blood pressure, but there is no threshold below which differences in blood pressure have no influence on risk. Nevertheless, practical people require a case definition, even if somewhat arbitrary, as a basis for decisions. An operational definition might be based on a threshold for treatment. This will take into account symptoms and prognosis but will not be determined consistently by either. A person may be symptom free yet benefit from treatment or alternatively may have an increased risk that cannot be remedied.

Each of these four approaches to case definition is suitable for a different purpose, so an investigator may need to define the purposes before cases can be defined.

Whatever approach is adopted, the case definition should as far as possible be precise and unambiguous. A standard textbook of cardiology proposes these electrocardiographic criteria for left bundle branch block: "The duration of QRS *commonly* measures 0·12 to 0·16 seconds . . . $V_5$ or $V_6$ exhibits a *large widened* R wave . . ." (*our italics*). As a basis for epidemiological comparisons this is potentially disastrous, because each investigator could interpret the italicised words differently. By contrast, the epidemiological "Minnesota Code" defines it like this: "QRS duration $\geqslant 0·12$ seconds in any one or more limb leads *and* R peak duration $\geqslant 0·06$ seconds in any one or more of leads, I, II, aVL, $V_5$, or $V_6$; each criterion to be met in a majority of technically adequate beats." If different studies are to be compared, case definitions must be rigorously standardised and free from ambiguity. Conventional clinical descriptions do not meet this requirement.

It is also essential to define and standardise the methods of measuring the chosen criteria. An important feature in diagnosing rheumatoid arthritis, for example, is early morning stiffness of the fingers; but two interviewers may emerge with different prevalence estimates if one takes an ordinary clinical history whereas the other uses a standard questionnaire. Cases in a survey are defined not by theoretical criteria, but in terms of response to specific investigative techniques. These, too, need to be defined, standardised, and reported adequately. As a result, epidemiological case definitions are narrower and more rigid than clinical ones. This loss of flexibility has to be accepted as the price of standardisation.

## Measures of disease frequency

For epidemiological purposes the occurrence of cases of disease must be related to the "population at risk" giving rise to the cases. Several measures of disease frequency are in common use.

### Incidence

The incidence of a disease is the *rate at which new cases occur in a population during a specified period*. For example, the incidence of thyrotoxicosis during 1982 was 10/100 000/year in Barrow-in-Furness compared with 49/100 000/year in Chester.

When the population at risk is roughly constant, incidence is measured as:

$$\frac{\textit{Number of new cases}}{\textit{Population at risk} \times \textit{time during which cases were ascertained}}$$

Sometimes measurement of incidence is complicated by changes in the population at risk during the period when cases are ascertained, for example, through births, deaths, or migrations. This difficulty is overcome by relating the numbers of new cases to the *person years at risk*, calculated by adding together the periods during which each individual member of the population is at risk during the measurement period. Thus incidence is defined as:

$$\frac{Number\ of\ new\ cases}{Total\ person\ years\ at\ risk}$$

It should be noted that once a person is classified as a case, he or she is no longer liable to become a new case, and therefore should not contribute further person years at risk. Sometimes the same pathological event happens more than once to the same individual. In the course of a study, a patient may have several episodes of myocardial infarction. In these circumstances the definition of incidence is usually restricted to the first event, although sometimes (for example in the study of infectious diseases) it is more appropriate to count all episodes. When ambiguity is possible reports should state whether incidence refers only to first diagnosis or to all episodes, as this may influence interpretation. For example, gonorrhoea notification rates in England and Wales increased dramatically during the 1960s, but no one knows to what extent this was due to more people getting infected or to the same people getting infected more often.

*Prevalence*

The prevalence of a disease is the *proportion of a population that are cases at a point in time*. The prevalence of persistent wheeze in a large sample of British primary school children surveyed during 1986 was approximately 3 per cent, the symptom being defined by response to a standard questionnaire completed by the children's parents. Prevalence is an appropriate measure only in such relatively stable conditions, and it is unsuitable for acute disorders.

Even in a chronic disease, the manifestations are often intermittent. In consequence, a "point" prevalence, based on a single examination, at one point in time, tends to underestimate the condition's total frequency. If repeated or continuous assessments of the same individuals are possible, a better measure is the *period prevalence* defined as *the proportion of a population that are cases at any time within a stated period.* Thus, the 12 month period prevalence of low back pain in a sample of British women aged 30–39 was found to be 33·6%.

## Mortality

Mortality is the *incidence of death from a disease.*

### Interrelation of incidence, prevalence, and mortality

Each new (incident) case enters a prevalence pool and remains there until either recovery or death:

$$\text{Incidence} \rightarrow \text{prevalence} \left\{ \begin{array}{l} \rightarrow recovery \\ \rightarrow death \end{array} \right.$$

If recovery and death rates are low, then chronicity is high and even a low incidence will produce a high prevalence:

$$Prevalence = incidence \times average\ duration$$

In studies of aetiology, incidence is the most appropriate measure of disease frequency. Mortality is a satisfactory proxy for incidence if survival is not related to the risk factors under investigation. However, patterns of mortality can be misleading if survival is variable. A recent decline in mortality from testicular cancer is attributable to improved cure rates from better treatment, and does not reflect a fall in incidence.

Prevalence is often used as an alternative to incidence in the study of rarer chronic diseases such as multiple sclerosis, where it would be difficult to accumulate large numbers of incident cases. Again, however, care is needed in interpretation. Differences in prevalence between different parts of the world may result from differences in survival and recovery as well as in incidence.

## Crude and specific rates

A crude incidence, prevalence, or mortality (death rate) is one that relates to results for a population taken as a whole, without subdivision or refinement. The crude mortality from lung cancer in men in England and Wales during 1985–89 was 1034/million/ year compared with 575/million/year during 1950–54. However, this bald fact masks a more complex pattern of trends in which

10

mortality from lung cancer was declining in younger men while going up in the elderly (fig).

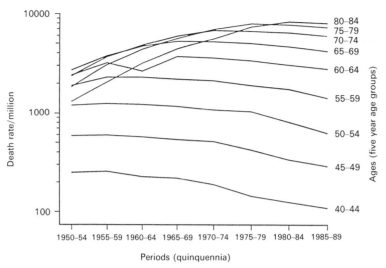

*Mortality from lung cancer in men in England and Wales, 1950–89, by five year age groups*

It is often helpful to break down results for the whole population to give rates specific for age and sex, but it is frustrating if results are given for 35–44 years in one report, 30–49 in another, and 31 to 40 in another. When feasible, decade classes should be 5–14, 15–24, and so on, and quinquennia should be 5–9, 10–14, and so on. Overlapping classes (5–10, 10–15) should be avoided.

## Extensions and alternatives to incidence and prevalence

The terms incidence and prevalence have been defined in relation to the onset and presence of disease, but they can be extended to encompass other events and states. Thus, one can measure the incidence of redundancy in an employed population (the rate at which people are made redundant over time) or the prevalence of smoking in it (the proportion of the population who currently smoke).

Some health outcomes do not lend themselves to description by

11

an incidence or prevalence, because of difficulties in defining the population at risk. For these outcomes, special rates are defined with a quasi population at risk as denominator.

---

SOME SPECIAL RATES

Birth rate

$$\frac{\text{Number of live births}}{\text{Mid-year population}}$$

Fertility rate

$$\frac{\text{Number of live births}}{\text{Number of women aged 15–44 years}}$$

Infant mortality rate

$$\frac{\text{Number of infant ( < 1 year) deaths}}{\text{Number of live births}}$$

Stillbirth rate

$$\frac{\text{Number of intrauterine deaths after 28 weeks}}{\text{Total births}}$$

Perinatal mortality rate

$$\frac{\text{Number of stillbirths + deaths in 1st week of life}}{\text{Total births}}$$

NB These rates are usually related to one year

---

Sometimes the population at risk can be satisfactorily defined, but it cannot be enumerated. For example, a cancer registry might collect information about the occupations of registered cancer cases, but not have data on the number of people in each occupation within its catchment area. Thus, the incidence of different cancers by occupation could not be calculated. An alternative in these circumstances would be to derive the proportion of different types of cancer in each occupational group. However, care is needed in the interpretation of proportions. A high proportion of prostatic cancers in farmers could reflect a high incidence of the disease, but it could also occur if farmers had an unusually low incidence of other types of cancer. Incidence and prevalence are preferable to proportions if they can be adequately measured.

# 3: Comparing disease rates

"Is this disease increasing in incidence? Does it occur with undue frequency in my local community? Does its incidence correlate with some suspected cause? Has the outcome changed since control measures were instituted?" To answer such questions means setting two sets of rates side by side and making some sense of the comparison. This chapter examines some of the problems that may arise.

## Terminology and classifications of disease

Diagnostic labels and groupings are many and various, and in continual flux: in the interests of communication some standardisation is necessary, even though no single system can meet all requirements.

*The ICD system*

The *International Classification of Diseases, Injuries, and Causes of Death*, published by the World Health Organisation, assigns a three character alphanumeric code to every major condition. Often a fourth character is added for more exact specification: for example, ICD C92 is "myeloid leukaemia", which may additionally be specified as C92·0 ("acute") or C92·1 ("chronic"). Broader groupings are readily formed—for example, ICD C81–C96 consists of all malignant neoplasms of lymphatic and haematopoietic tissue. This system is used for coding death certificates. It determines the presentation of results in the registrar general's reports and in the diagnostic registers of most hospitals.

The system has to be revised periodically to keep pace with medical usage. The ninth revision came into general use in 1979, and has now been superseded by the 10th revision for many applications. When the classification alters from one revision to the next, disease rates may not be directly comparable before and after the change. For example, the eighth revision included separate categories for gastric ulcer and for peptic ulcer of unspecified sites, whereas in the seventh revision this distinction was not made. In this situation some aggregation of categories is needed before valid comparisons can be made.

## Measures of association

Several measures are commonly used to summarise comparisons of disease rates between populations, each with its special applications. The definitions given here assume that rates in an "exposed" population are being compared with those in "unexposed" people. The exposure might be to "risk factors" suspected of causing the disease (for example, being bottle fed or owning a cat) or of protecting against it (for example, immunisation). Parallel definitions can be used to compare disease rates between people with different levels of exposure to a risk factor (for example, people with high or low aluminium concentrations in their drinking water).

*Attributable risk* is the disease rate in exposed persons minus that in unexposed persons. It is the measure of association that is most relevant when making decisions for individuals. For example, in deciding whether or not to indulge in a dangerous sport such as rock climbing, it is the attributable risk of injury which must be weighed against the pleasures of participation.

*Relative risk* is the ratio of the disease rate in exposed persons to that in people who are unexposed. It is related to attributable risk by the formula:

*Attributable risk = rate of disease in unexposed persons × (relative risk − 1)*

Relative risk is less relevant to making decisions in risk management than is attributable risk. For example, given a choice between a doubling in their risk of death from bronchial carcinoma and a doubling in their risk of death from oral cancer, most informed people would opt for the latter. The relative risk is the same (two), but the corresponding attributable risk is lower because oral cancer is a rarer disease. Nevertheless, relative risk is the measure of association most often used by epidemiologists. One reason for this is that it can be estimated by a wider range of study designs. In particular, relative risk can be estimated from case-control studies (see chapter 8) whereas attributable risk cannot. Another reason is the empirical observation that where two risk factors for a disease act in concert, their relative risks often come close to multiplying. Table I shows risks of lung cancer in smokers and non-smokers according to whether or not they had worked with asbestos. Risk in smokers was about 10-fold more than in non-smokers, irrespective of exposure to asbestos. Attributable risk does not show this convenient invariance as often as relative risk.

TABLE I—*Relative risks of lung cancer according to smoking habits and exposure to asbestos*

| Exposure to asbestos | Cigarette smoking | |
|---|---|---|
| | No | Yes |
| No | 1·0 | 10·9 |
| Yes | 5·2 | 53·2 |

Closely related to relative risk is the *odds ratio*, defined as the odds of disease in exposed persons divided by the odds of disease in unexposed persons. People who bet on horses will be aware that a rate or chance of one in 100 corresponds to odds of 99 to one against; and in general a rate of one in $x$ is equivalent to odds of one to $x-1$. In most circumstances, the odds ratio is a close approximation to relative risk.

*Population attributable risk* is the rate of disease in a population minus the rate that would apply if all of the population were unexposed. It is related to attributable risk by the formula:

$$\text{Population attributable} = \text{attributable} \times \text{prevalence of exposure to}$$
$$\text{risk} \qquad\qquad \text{risk} \qquad\qquad \text{risk factor in population}$$

Population attributable risk measures the potential impact of control measures in a population, and is relevant to decisions in public health.

*Attributable proportion* is the proportion of disease that would be eliminated in a population if its disease rate were reduced to that of unexposed persons. It is used to compare the potential impact of different public health strategies.

## Confounding

In an ideal laboratory experiment the investigator alters only one variable at a time, so that any effect he observes can only be due to that variable. Most epidemiological studies are observational, not experimental, and compare people who differ in all kinds of ways, known and unknown. If such differences determine risk of disease independently of the exposure under investigation, they are said to *confound* its association with the disease.

For example, several studies have indicated high rates of lung cancer in cooks. Though this could be a consequence of their work (perhaps caused by carcinogens in fumes from frying), it may be simply because professional cooks smoke more than the average. In other words, smoking might confound the association with cooking.

Confounding determines the extent to which observed associations are causal. It may give rise to spurious associations when in fact there is no causal relation, or at the other extreme, it may obscure the effects of a true cause.

Two common confounding factors are age and sex. Crude mortality from all causes in males over a five year period was higher in Bournemouth than in Southampton. However, this difference disappeared when death rates were compared for specific age groups (table II). It occurred not because Bournemouth is a less healthy place than Southampton but because, being a town to which people retire, it has a more elderly population.

## Standardisation

The above example shows the dangers of drawing aetiological conclusions from comparisons of crude rates. The problem can be overcome by comparing age and sex specific rates as in table II, but the presentation of such data is rather cumbersome, and it is often helpful to derive a single statistic that summarises the comparison while allowing for differences in the age and sex structure of the

TABLE II—*Deaths in males in Bournemouth and Southampton during a five year period*

| Age group (years) | Bournemouth | | | Southampton | | |
|---|---|---|---|---|---|---|
| | No of deaths | Population | Annual death rate per 100 000 | No of deaths | Population | Annual death rate per 100 000 |
| <1 | 116 | 919 | 2 524 | 223 | 1 897 | 2 351 |
| 1–44 | 204 | 34 616 | 118 | 332 | 64 090 | 104 |
| 45–64 | 1 252 | 19 379 | 1 292 | 1 728 | 24 440 | 1 414 |
| 65 + | 4 076 | 11 760 | 6 932 | 3 639 | 9 120 | 7 980 |
| All ages | 5 648 | 66 674 | 1 694 | 5 922 | 99 547 | 1 190 |

populations under study. *Standardised* or *adjusted rates* provide for this need. Two techniques are available:

## Direct standardisation

Direct standardisation entails comparison of weighted averages of age and sex specific disease rates, the weights being equal to the proportion' of people in each age and sex group in a convenient reference population. Table III shows the method of calculation, based on mortality from coronary heart disease in men in the USA aged 35–64 during 1968. Table IV gives standardised rates for men and women in the ensuing years, calculated in the same way, and shows a remarkable fall.

TABLE III—*Example of direct standardisation, based on mortality from coronary heart disease (CHD) in men in the USA aged 35–64, 1968*

| Age (years) | CHD deaths/100 000 (1) | % of reference population in age group (2) | (1) × (2) |
|---|---|---|---|
| 35–44 | 93 | 34·4 | 3 199·2 |
| 45–54 | 355 | 36·0 | 12 780·0 |
| 55–64 | 961 | 29·5 | 28 349·5 |
| Total | | 100 | 44 328·7 ÷ 100 = 443 |

TABLE IV—*Coronary heart disease in American men and women aged 35–64: changes in age standardised mortality (deaths/100 000/year) during 1968–74*

|       | 1968 | 1969 | 1970 | 1971 | 1972 | 1973 | 1974 |
|-------|------|------|------|------|------|------|------|
| Men   | 443  | 430  | 420  | 413  | 408  | 399  | 377  |
| Women | 134  | 126  | 126  | 124  | 120  | 118  | 111  |

## Indirect standardisation

The direct method is for large studies, and in most surveys the indirect method yields more stable risk estimates. Suppose that a general practitioner wants to test his impression of a local excess of chronic bronchitis. Using a standard questionnaire, he examines a sample of middle aged men from his list, and finds that 45 have persistent cough and phlegm. Is this excessive? The calculation is shown in table V.

TABLE V—*Example of indirect standardisation*

| Age (years) | No in study (1) | Symptom prevalence in reference group (2) | Expected cases = (1) × (2) |
|-------------|-----------------|-------------------------------------------|-----------------------------|
| 35–44       | 150             | 8%                                        | 12                          |
| 45–54       | 100             | 9%                                        | 9                           |
| 55–64       | 90              | 10%                                       | 9                           |
| Total       |                 |                                           | 30                          |

First the numbers of subjects in each age class are listed (column 1). The doctor must then choose a suitable reference population in which the class specific rates are known (column 2). (In mortality studies this would usually be the nation or some subset of it, such as a particular region or social class; in multicentre studies it could be the pooled data from all centres.) Cross multiplying columns 1 and 2 for each class gives the expected *number* of cases in a group of that age and size, based on the reference population's rates. Summation over all classes yields the total expected frequency, given the size and age structure of that particular study sample. Where 30 cases were expected he has observed 45, giving an age adjusted *relative risk* or *standardised prevalence ratio* of

45/30 = 150%. (Conventionally, standardised ratios are often expressed as percentages.)

A comparable statistic, the *standardised mortality ratio* (SMR) is widely used by the registrar general in summarising time trends and regional and occupational differences. Thus in 1981 the standardised mortality ratio for death by suicide in male doctors was 172%, indicating a large excess relative to the general population at the time. To analyse time trends, as with the cost of living index, an arbitrary base year is taken.

## Other methods of adjusting for confounders

The techniques of standardisation are usually used to adjust for age and sex, although they can be applied to control for other confounders. Other methods, which are used more generally to adjust for confounding, include mathematical modelling techniques such as *logistic regression*. These assume that a person's risk of disease is a specified mathematical function of his exposure to different risk factors and confounders. For example, it might be assumed that his odds of developing lung cancer are a product of a constant and three parameters—one determined by his age, one by whether he smokes, and the third by whether he has worked with asbestos. A computer program is then used to calculate the values of the parameters that best fit the observed data. These parameters estimate the odds ratios for each risk factor—age, smoking, and exposure to asbestos, and are mutually adjusted. Such modelling techniques are powerful and readily available to users of personal computers. They should be used with caution, however, as the mathematical assumptions in the model may not always reflect the realities of biology.

19

# 4: Measurement error and bias

Epidemiological studies measure characteristics of populations. The parameter of interest may be a disease rate, the prevalence of an exposure, or more often some measure of the association between an exposure and disease. Because studies are carried out on people and have all the attendant practical and ethical constraints, they are almost invariably subject to *bias*.

Bias is a systematic tendency to underestimate or overestimate the parameter of interest because of a deficiency in the design or execution of a study. Many sources of bias in epidemiological studies have been distinguished, but two main classes will be considered here.

## Selection bias

Selection bias occurs when the subjects studied are not representative of the target population about which conclusions are to be drawn. Suppose that an investigator wishes to estimate the prevalence of heavy alcohol consumption (more than 21 units a week) in adult residents of a city. He might try to do this by selecting a random sample from all the adults registered with local general practitioners, and sending them a postal questionnaire about their drinking habits. With this design, one source of error would be the exclusion from the study sample of those residents not registered with a doctor. These excluded subjects might have different patterns of drinking from those included in the study. Also, not all of the subjects selected for study will necessarily complete and return questionnaires, and non-responders may have different drinking habits from those who take the trouble to reply. Both of these deficiences are potential sources of selection bias. The possibility of selection bias should always be considered when defining a study sample. Furthermore, when responses are incomplete, the scope for bias must be assessed. The problems of incomplete response to surveys are considered further in chapter 5.

## Information bias

The other major class of bias arises from errors in measuring exposure or disease. In a study to estimate the relative risk of congenital malformations associated with maternal exposure to organic solvents such as white spirit, mothers of malformed babies were questioned about their contact with such substances during pregnancy, and their answers were compared with those from control mothers with normal babies. With this design there was a danger that "case" mothers, who were highly motivated to find out why their babies had been born with an abnormality, might recall past exposure more completely than controls. If so, a bias would result with a tendency to exaggerate risk estimates.

Another study looked at risk of hip osteoarthritis according to physical activity at work, cases being identified from records of admission to hospital for hip replacement. Here there was a possibility of bias because subjects with physically demanding jobs might be more handicapped by a given level of arthritis and therefore seek treatment more readily.

Bias cannot usually be totally eliminated from epidemiological studies. The aim, therefore, must be to keep it to a minimum, to identify those biases that cannot be avoided, to assess their potential impact, and to take this into account when interpreting results. The motto of the epidemiologist could well be "dirty hands but a clean mind" (*manus sordidae, mens pura*).

## Measurement error

As indicated above, errors in measuring exposure or disease can be an important source of bias in epidemiological studies In conducting studies, therefore, it is important to assess the quality of measurements. An ideal survey technique is valid (that is, it measures accurately what it purports to measure). Sometimes a reliable standard is available against which the validity of a survey method can be assessed. For example, a sphygmomanometer's validity can be measured by comparing its readings with intra-arterial pressures, and the validity of a mammographic diagnosis of breast cancer can be tested (if the woman agrees) by biopsy. More often, however, there is no sure reference standard. The validity of a questionnaire for diagnosing angina cannot be fully known: clinical opinion varies among experts, and even coronary arteriograms may be normal in true cases or abnormal in symptomless people. The pathologist can describe changes at necropsy, but these may say little about the patient's symptoms or functional state. Measurements of disease in life are often incapable of full validation.

In practice, therefore, validity may have to be assessed indirectly. Two approaches are used commonly. A technique that has been simplified and standardised to make it suitable for use in surveys may be compared with the best conventional clinical assessment. A self administered psychiatric questionnaire, for instance, may be compared with the majority opinion of a psychiatric panel. Alternatively, a measurement may be validated by its ability to predict future illness. Validation by predictive ability may, however, require the study of many subjects.

## Analysing validity

When a survey technique or test is used to dichotomise subjects (for example, as cases or non-cases, exposed or not exposed) its validity is analysed by classifying subjects as positive or negative, firstly by the survey method and secondly according to the standard reference test. The findings can then be expressed in a contingency table as shown on page 23:

From this table four important statistics can be derived:

*Sensitivity*—A sensitive test detects a high proportion of the true cases, and this quality is measured here by $a/a + c$.

*Specificity*—A specific test has few false positives, and this quality is measured by $d/b + d$.

*Systematic error*—For epidemiological rates it is particularly important for the test to give the right total count of cases. This is measured by the ratio of the total numbers positive to the survey and the reference tests, or $(a + b)/(a + c)$.

*Predictive value*—This is the proportion of positive test results

TABLE I—*Comparison of a survey test with a reference test*

| Survey test result | Reference test result | | |
|---|---|---|---|
| | Positive | Negative | Totals |
| Positive | True positives, correctly identified = (a) | False positives = (b) | Total test positives = (a + b) |
| Negative | False negatives = (c) | True negatives correctly identified = (d) | Total test negatives = (c + d) |
| Totals | Total true positives = (a + c) | Total true negatives = (b + d) | Grand total = (a + b + c + d) |

that are truly positive. It is important in screening, and will be discussed further in chapter 10.

It should be noted that both systematic error and predictive value depend on the relative frequency of true positives and true negatives in the study sample (that is, on the prevalence of the disease or exposure that is being measured).

## Sensitive or specific? A matter of choice

If the criteria for a positive test result are stringent then there will be few false positives but the test will be insensitive. Conversely, if criteria are relaxed then there will be fewer false negatives but the test will be less specific. In a survey of breast cancer alternative diagnostic criteria were compared with the results of a reference test (biopsy). Clinical palpation by a doctor yielded fewest false positives (93% specificity), but missed half the cases (50% sensitivity). Criteria for diagnosing "a case" were then relaxed to include all the positive results identified by doctor's palpation, nurse's palpation, or *x* ray mammography: few cases were then missed (94% sensitivity), but specificity fell to 86%.

By choosing the right test and cut off points it may be possible to get the balance of sensitivity and specificity that is best for a particular study. In a survey to establish prevalence this might be when false positives balance false negatives. In a study to compare rates in different populations the absolute rates are less important, the primary concern being to avoid systematic bias in the comparisons: a specific test may well be preferred, even at the price of some loss of sensitivity.

## Repeatability

When there is no satisfactory standard against which to assess the validity of a measurement technique, then examining its repeatability is often helpful. Consistent findings do not necessarily imply that the technique is valid: a laboratory test may yield persistently false positive results, or a very repeatable psychiatric questionnaire may be an insensitive measure of, for example, "stress". However, poor repeatability indicates either poor validity or that the characteristic that is being measured varies over time. In either of these circumstances results must be interpreted with caution.

Repeatability can be tested within observers (that is, the same observer performing the measurement on two separate occasions) and also between observers (comparing measurements made by different observers on the same subject or specimen). Assessment of repeatability may be built into a study—a sample of people undergoing a second examination or a sample of radiographs, blood samples, and so on being tested in duplicate. Even a small sample is valuable, provided that (1) it is representative and (2) the duplicate tests are genuinely independent. If testing is done "off line" (perhaps as part of a pilot study) then particular care is needed to ensure that subjects, observers, and operating conditions are all adequately representative of the main study. It is much easier to test repeatability when material can be transported and stored—for example, deep frozen plasma samples, histological sections, and all kinds of tracings and photographs. However, such tests may exclude an important source of observer variation—namely the techniques of obtaining samples and records.

## Reasons for variation in replicate measurements

Independent replicate measurements in the same subjects are usually found to vary more than one's gloomiest expectations. To interpret the results, and to seek remedies, it is helpful to dissect the total variability into its four components:

*Within observer variation*—Discovering one's own inconsistency can be traumatic; it highlights a lack of clear criteria of measurement and interpretation, particularly in dealing with the grey area between "normal" and "abnormal". It is largely *random*—that is, unpredictable in direction.

*Between observer variation*—This includes the first component (the instability of individual observers), but adds to it an extra and *systematic* component due to individual differences in techniques and criteria. Unfortunately, this may be large in relation to the real difference between groups that it is hoped to identify. It may be possible to avoid this problem, either by using a single observer or, if material is transportable, by forwarding it all for central examination. Alternatively, the bias within a survey may be neutralised by random allocation of subjects to observers. Each observer should be identified by a code number on the survey record; analysis of results by observer will then indicate any major problems, and perhaps permit some statistical correction for the bias.

*Random subject variation*—When measured repeatedly in the same person, physiological variables like blood pressure tend to show a roughly normal distribution around the subject's mean. Nevertheless, surveys usually have to make do with a single measurement, and the imprecision will not be noticed unless the extent of subject variation has been studied. Random subject variation has some important implications for screening and also in clinical practice, when people with extreme initial values are recalled. Thanks to a statistical quirk this group then seems to improve because its members include some whose mean value is normal but who by chance had higher values at first examination: on average, their follow up values necessarily tend to fall (*regression to the mean*). The size of this effect depends on the amount of random subject variation. Misinterpretation can be avoided by repeat examinations to establish an adequate baseline, or (in an intervention study) by including a control group.

*Biased (systematic) subject variation*—Blood pressure is much influenced by the temperature of the examination room, as well as by less readily standardised emotional factors. Surveys to detect diabetes find a much higher prevalence in the afternoon than in the morning; and the standard bronchitis questionnaire possibly elicits more positive responses in winter than in summer. Thus conditions and timing of an investigation may have a major effect on an individual's true state and on his or her responses. As far as possible, studies should be designed to control for this—for example, by testing for diabetes at one time of day. Alternatively, a variable such as room temperature can be measured and allowed for in the analysis.

## Analysing repeatability

The repeatability of measurements of continuous numerical variables such as blood pressure can be summarised by the *standard deviation* of replicate measurements or by their *coefficient of variation* (standard deviation ÷ mean). When pairs of measurements have been made, either by the same observer on two different occasions or by two different observers, a scatter plot will conveniently show the extent and pattern of observer variation.

For qualitative attributes, such as clinical symptoms and signs, the results are first set out as a contingency table:

TABLE II—*Comparison of results obtained by two observers*

|  |  | Observer 1 | |
|---|---|---|---|
|  |  | Positive | Negative |
| Observer 2 | Positive | a | b |
|  | Negative | c | d |

The overall level of agreement could be represented by the proportion of the total in cells a and d. This measure unfortunately turns out to depend more on the prevalence of the condition than on the repeatability of the method. This is because in practice it is easy to agree on a straightforward negative; disagreements depend on the prevalence of the difficult borderline cases. Instead, therefore, repeatability is usually summarised by the $\kappa$ *statistic*, which measures the level of agreement over and above what would be expected from the prevalence of the attribute.

# 5: Planning and conducting a survey

Epidemiological surveys use various study designs and range widely in size. At one extreme a case-control investigation may include fewer than 50 subjects, while at the other, some large longitudinal studies follow up many thousands of people for several decades. The main study designs will be described in later chapters, but we here discuss important features that are common to the planning and execution of surveys, whatever their specific design.

## Early planning

The success of data collection requires careful preparation. The first and often the most difficult question is "Why am I doing this survey?" Many studies start with a general hope that something interesting will emerge, and they often end in frustration. The general interest has first to be translated into precisely formulated, written objectives. Every survey should be reasonably sure to give an adequate answer to at least one specific question. This initial planning requires some idea of the final analysis; and it may be useful at the outset to outline the key tables for the final report, and to consider the numbers of cases expected in their major cells.

Every study needs a primary purpose. It is easy to argue "While we have the subjects there, let's also measure . . ."; but overloading, whether of investigators or subjects, must be avoided if it in any way threatens the primary purpose. Sometimes subsidiary objectives may be pursued in subsamples (every nth subject, or in a particular age group) or by recalling some subjects for a second examination: when their initial contact has been favourable then response to recall is usually good.

*Background reading*

Before planning the detail of a study, it is wise to carry out a library search of the relevant background publications. Occasionally this may show the answer to the study question without any need for further data collection; or it may uncover useful sources of published information, such as the registrar general's mortality and cancer registry reports, which can form the basis of an analysis without the requirement for an expensive and time consuming field survey. Even when survey work remains necessary, experience in earlier related investigations may guide the design or indicate pitfalls to be avoided.

## Choice of examination methods

The overriding need in an epidemiological survey is to examine a representative sample of adequate size in a standardised and sufficiently valid way. This determines the choice of examination methods and the points where these differ from those of clinical practice. Methods must be acceptable, and if possible non-invasive, or else cooperation suffers and the study group becomes unrepresentative. They must be relatively cheap and quick, or not enough subjects can be examined: with fixed resources the need for detail conflicts with the need for numbers. Most important of all, methods and observers must be capable of rigorous standardisation; even if this excludes the benefits of clinical judgement.

*Information abstracted from existing records*

Sometimes adequately standardised information is already available from existing records. For example, in a study to examine the long term incidence of hypothyroidism after treatment with radioiodine for thyrotoxicosis, it was possible to identify treated patients and obtain the information needed to follow them up (name, date of birth, sex, address, etc) by searching hospital files. When existing records are exploited in this way, the required information is normally abstracted on to a specially designed form or even direct on to a portable computer.

The design of the abstraction form or of the computer program for inputting data should take into account the layout of the source material. Having to flick repeatedly backwards and forwards through the source record is not only tedious and time consuming, but may also increase the chance of error. Each abstracted record should be identified by a serial number, and should include sufficient information to permit easy access back to the source material for checking and to obtain additional data if required. When data are not abstracted direct on to computer, later transfer to computer will often be facilitated by numerical coding, in which case coding boxes can be provided on the right hand side of the abstraction form. Some items of data (for example, dates of birth) can easily be written direct into the coding boxes. Others, such as occupation, may need to be recorded in words and coded later as a separate exercise. Time spent writing is minimised if non-numerical information is, when possible, ringed or ticked rather than having to be written out. To minimise the chance of error, any reformulation of numerical data (for example, derivation of age at hospital admission from date of birth and date of admission) should be carried out by the computer after date entry, and not as part of the abstraction process. When coding data, allowance must be made for the possibility of missing information.

*Questionnaires*

Epidemiological data are often obtained by means of question-naires. These may be either self administered (that is, completed by the subject) or administered at interview. Self administered questionnaires are easier to standardise because the possibility of systematic differences in interviewing technique is avoided. On the other hand, they are limited by the need to be unambiguously understood by all subjects. An interviewer may be essential to collect information on complex topics.

Good design of questionnaires requires skill. The language used should be clear and simple. Two short questions, each covering one point, are better than one longer question which covers two points at once. A question that has been used successfully in a previous study has obvious advantages. The order of questions should take into account the sensitivities of the person to whom they are addressed—it is better to start with "What is your date of birth?" than launch straight into "Have you ever been treated for gonorrhoea?"—and should be designed to facilitate recall. For example, all questions relating to one phase of the person's life might be grouped together. As a check on the reliability of

29

information, it may sometimes be helpful to include overlapping questions. In a study of risk factors for back pain, some people reported that their jobs entailed driving for more than four hours a day but did not involve more than two hours sitting. This suggests that they had not properly understood the questions. An important consideration is whether to use closed or open ended questions. Closed ended questions, with one box for each possible answer (including "don't know") are more readily answered and classified, but cannot always collect information in the detail that is required. When interviewers are used then the wording with which they ask questions should be standardised as far as is compatible with the need to obtain useful information. As in abstracting existing records, the forms used to record answers to questions should be designed for ease and accuracy of completion and to simplify subsequent coding and analysis.

*Physical examination and clinical investigations*

Methods of physical examination should be designed to reduce variation within and between observers. Often, a quantitative measurement (for example, respiratory rate) is easier to standardise than a qualitative judgement (whether someone is tachypnoeic or not). Standardisation of laboratory assays can be improved by careful specification of the method by which specimens should be collected and stored and by rigorous quality control of the analysis.

Whatever method of data collection is adopted, it is usually worth trying it out in a pilot survey before embarking on the main study. Identification of practical snags at this stage can save much difficulty later. In large studies the questionnaire or record design should be discussed with the statistician who will later be concerned in the analysis.

## Staff and training

In a small study the doctor himself may do all the work, but in large surveys he will need helpers. If an epidemiological examination technique requires skill and clinical judgement it has probably been insufficiently standardised: if it is adequately standardised it can usually be taught to any intelligent person.

The figure shows how two observers had distinct but opposite time trends in their performances during the early stages of a survey of skinfold thickness. Such training effects, which are common, should have been completed before the start of the main study:

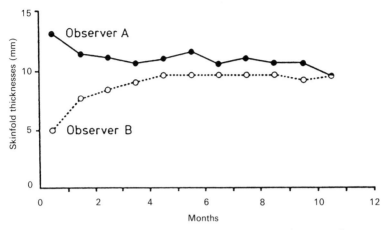

*Trend in mean values for triceps skinfold thickness obtained by two observers in the same survey*

new staff need supervised practice under realistic field conditions followed by pre-survey testing.

Despite all precautions, observer differences may persist. Observers should therefore be allocated to subjects in a more or less random way: if, for example, one person examined most of the men, and another most of the women, then observer differences would be confounded with true sex differences. To maintain quality control throughout the survey each examiner's identity should be entered on the record, and results for different examiners may then be compared.

## Sampling

### Sample size

Most surveys and trials are smaller than the investigator would wish, lack of numbers often setting a limit to some desirable subgroup analysis. This is inevitable. What can be avoided is discovering only at the final analysis that numbers do not permit achievement even of the study's primary objective. To prevent this

31

disappointment the purpose of the study has first to be formulated in precise statistical terms. If the aim is to estimate prevalence, then sample size will depend on the required accuracy of that estimate. (The table gives some examples.) Sampling error is proportionally greater for less common conditions; that is to say, to achieve the same level of confidence requires a larger sample if prevalence is low.

*95% confidence limits for various rates and sample sizes*

| Estimated prevalence (%) | 95% confidence limits | |
|---|---|---|
| | n = 500 | n = 1000 |
| 2 | 1·0–3·7 | 1·2–3·1 |
| 10 | 7·5–13·0 | 8·2–12·0 |
| 20 | 16·6–23·8 | 17·6–22·6 |

Techniques also exist for calculating sample sizes required for estimating, with specified precision, the mean value of a variable, or for identifying a given difference in prevalence or mean values between two populations. These techniques may be found in textbooks or (better) by consulting a statistician; but either way the investigators must first know exactly what they want to achieve.

*Sampling methods*

When the study sample is selected from a larger study population, statistical inference will be more rigorous if the selection process is random, or effectively random; that is to say, if each individual in the study population has a known (usually identical) non-zero probability of selection. To achieve this a *census* or listing of the study population is first required. In a survey of adults in a hospital district the electoral register will probably serve. In an occupational group the payroll is invariably complete, and in a school there are class registers. In general practice there is an age-sex register. To choose a *simple random sample* the listed people are numbered serially. Numbers within the appropriate range are then read off from a table or computer generated list of random numbers until enough people have been selected.

It may be that an investigator wishes to choose a sample in which certain subgroups (particular ages, for instance, or high risk categories) are relatively overrepresented. To achieve this he may divide the study population into subgroups (*strata*) and then draw a separate random sample from each, while adjusting the various sample sizes to suit the investigation's requirements. This is a *stratified random sample*.

The study population may be large and widely scattered—for example, all the general practices in a city—but for the sake of convenience the investigator may wish to concentrate his survey in a few areas only. This can be done by drawing first a random sample of practices, and then, within these practices, drawing a random sample of individuals. Such *two stage sampling* works well, but there is some loss of statistical efficiency, especially if only a few units are selected at the first stage.

## Recruiting subjects

Most people are willing to take part in medical surveys provided that they trust the investigators, just as patients will nearly always help their own doctors in their research. In population studies, however, there has usually been no previous contact. The selected subjects need an explanation of the purpose of the study, of why they in particular have been asked to take part, of what is expected from them, and what if anything they will get out of it (for instance a medical check up or a report on the research findings). Local general practitioners, too, need to know what is going on. Time given to preparatory public relations is always well spent.

Response must be made as easy as possible. If attendance at a centre is required, it is better to send everyone a provisional appointment than to expect them to reply to a letter asking whether they are willing to attend. Provision of transport may be welcomed. Often the difference between a mediocre response and a good one is tactful persistence, including second invitations (perhaps by recorded delivery), telephone calls, identifying the reasons for non-attendance, and home visits.

### Response rates

The level of response that is acceptable depends both on the study question and on the population in which the question is being asked. Problems arise because non-responders may be atypical. For example, in a survey of coronary risk factors among adults registered with a group practice, those at highest risk may be the least inclined to complete a questionnaire or attend for examination. If a response rate of 85% were achieved, an estimated prevalence of heavy alcohol consumption of 3% among the responders could be substantially too low if most of the non-responders drank heavily. On the other hand an estimated 50% prevalence of smokers would not need major revision, even if all of the non-responders smoked.

What matters is how unrepresentative non-responders are in relation to the study question. It is not important whether they are atypical in other respects. In a survey to evaluate the association between serum IgE concentrations and ventilatory function it would not matter if non-responders had an unusually high frequency of respiratory disease, provided that the relation of their ventilatory function to IgE was not unrepresentative.

Assessment of the likely bias resulting from incomplete response is ultimately a matter of judgement. However, two approaches may help the assessment. Firstly, a small random sample can be drawn from the non-responders, and particularly vigorous efforts made to encourage their participation, including home visits. The findings for this subsample will then indicate the extent of bias among non-responders as a whole. Secondly, some information is generally available for all people listed in the study population. From this it will be possible to contrast responders and non-responders with respect to characteristics such as age, sex, and residence. Differences will alert the investigator to the possibility of bias.

In addition, it may help to put absolute bounds on the uncertainty arising from non-response by making extreme assumptions about the non-responders. For example, if the aim of a survey were to estimate a disease prevalence, what would be the prevalence if all of the non-responders had the disease, or none of them?

## Analysis

Small studies can sometimes be analysed manually with the help of a calculator. Nowadays, however, the analysis of epidemiological data is almost always carried out by computer. With recent advances in technology, all but the largest data sets can be handled satisfactorily on a personal computer. Moreover, a wide range of software packages is now available to assist epidemiological analysis.

The starting point for analysis by computer is the coding and entry of data. These procedures should be checked, usually by carrying them out in duplicate. In addition, once the data have been entered, further checks should be made to ensure that all codes are valid (for example, nobody should have 31 February as a birth date) and to look for any internal inconsistencies (such as a date of admission to hospital being earlier than the subject's date of birth). Statistical analysis should only begin when the data set is as "clean" as possible.

With the ready availability of software packages, it is tempting for medical investigators to embark on analyses they do not fully understand, and in the process they may use inappropriate statistical techniques. For this reason it is preferable to obtain advice from a statistician when carrying out all but the simplest analyses. As with the earlier stages of data processing, statistical calculations should all be checked.

# 6: Ecological studies

Most epidemiological investigations of aetiology are observational. They look for associations between the occurrence of disease and exposure to known or suspected causes. In ecological studies the unit of observation is the population or community. Disease rates and exposures are measured in each of a series of populations and their relation is examined. Often the information about disease and exposure is abstracted from published statistics and therefore does not require expensive or time consuming data collection. The populations compared may be defined in various ways.

## Geographical comparisons

One common approach is to look for geographical correlations between disease incidence or mortality and the prevalence of risk factors. For example, mortality from coronary heart disease in local authority areas of England and Wales has been correlated with neonatal mortality in the same places 70 and more years earlier. This observation generated the hypothesis that coronary heart disease may result from the impaired development of blood vessels and other tissues in fetal life and infancy.

Many useful observations have emerged from geographical analyses, but care is needed in their interpretation. Allowance can be made for the potential confounding effects of age and sex by appropriate standardisation (see chapter 3). More troublesome, however, are the biases that can occur if ascertainment of disease or exposure, or both, differs from one place to another. For example, a survey of back disorders found a higher incidence of general practitioner consultation for back pain in the north than the south of Britain, which might suggest greater exposure to some causative agent or activity in the north. Closer investigation, however, indicated that the prevalence of back symptoms was similar in both regions and that it was patients' consultation habits that varied. Thus, in this instance correlations based on general practitioner consultation rates would be quite misleading. A study based on rates of admission to hospital for perforated peptic ulcer would probably be reliable as in affluent countries almost all cases will reach hospital and be diagnosed. On the other hand, unbiased ascertainment of disorders such as depression or Parkinson's disease may be difficult without a specially designed survey. When there is doubt about the uniformity of ascertainment, it may be necessary to explore the extent of any possible bias in a validation exercise.

## Time trends

Many diseases show remarkable fluctuations in incidence over time. Rates of acute infection can vary appreciably over a few days, but epidemics of chronic disorders such as lung cancer and coronary heart disease evolve over decades. If time or *secular* trends in disease incidence correlate with changes in a community's environment or way of life then the trends may provide important clues to aetiology. Thus, the currently increasing incidence of melanoma in Britain has been linked with greater exposure to sunlight (from fashions in dress and holidays abroad); and successive rises and falls in mortality from cervical cancer have been related to varying levels of sexual promiscuity, as evidenced by notification rates for gonorrhoea.

Like geographical studies, analysis of secular trends may be biased by differences in the ascertainment of disease. As health services have improved, diagnostic criteria and techniques have changed. Furthermore, whereas in geographical studies the differences are accessible to current inquiry, validating secular changes is more difficult as it depends on observations made and often scantily recorded many years ago. Nevertheless, the reality— if not the true size—of secular trends can often be established with reasonable certainty. The rise and subsequent fall in the incidence of appendicitis in Britain during the past 100 years is a good example.

## Migrants

The study of migrant populations offers a way of discriminating

37

genetic from environmental causes of geographical variation in disease, and may also indicate the age at which an environmental cause exerts its effect. Second generation Japanese migrants to the USA have substantially lower rates of stomach cancer than Japanese people in Japan, indicating that the high incidence of the disease in Japan is environmental in origin. In first generation migrants rates are intermediate, which suggests that the adverse environmental influences act, at least in part, early in life.

In interpreting migrant studies it is important to bear in mind the possibility that the migrants may be unrepresentative of the population that they leave, and that their health may have been affected directly by the process of migration. Norwegian immigrants into the USA, for example, have been found to have a higher incidence of psychosis than people in Norway. Although this may indicate environmental influences in the USA that led to psychotic illness, it may also have resulted from selective emigration from Norway of people more susceptible to mental illness, or from the unusual stresses imposed on immigrants during their adjustment to a foreign culture.

Despite these difficulties, migrant studies have contributed importantly to our understanding of several diseases.

## Occupation and social class

The other populations for whom statistics on disease incidence and mortality are readily available are occupational and socio-economic groups. Thus, mortality from pneumonia is high in welders, and the steep social class gradient in mortality from chronic obstructive lung disease is evidence that correlates of poverty, perhaps bad housing, have an important influence on the disease.

# 7: Longitudinal studies

In a longitudinal study subjects are followed over time with continuous or repeated monitoring of risk factors or health outcomes, or both. Such investigations vary enormously in their size and complexity. At one extreme a large population may be studied over decades. For example, the longitudinal study of the Office of Population Censuses and Surveys prospectively follows a 1% sample of the British population that was initially identified at the 1971 census. Outcomes such as mortality and incidence of cancer have been related to employment status, housing, and other variables measured at successive censuses. At the other extreme, some longitudinal studies follow up relatively small groups for a few days or weeks. Thus, firemen acutely exposed to noxious fumes might be monitored to identify any immediate effects.

Most longitudinal studies examine associations between exposure to known or suspected causes of disease and subsequent morbidity or mortality. In the simplest design a sample or *cohort* of subjects exposed to a risk factor is identified along with a sample of unexposed controls. The two groups are then followed up prospectively, and the incidence of disease in each is measured. By comparing the incidence rates, attributable and relative risks can be estimated. Allowance can be made for suspected confounding factors either by *matching* the controls to the exposed subjects so that they have a similar pattern of exposure to the confounder, or by measuring exposure to the confounder in each group and adjusting for any difference in the statistical analysis.

A problem when the cohort method is applied to the study

of chronic diseases such as cancer, coronary heart disease, or diabetes is that large numbers of people must be followed up for long periods before sufficient cases accrue to give statistically meaningful results. The difficulty is further increased when, as for example with most carcinogens, there is a long induction period between first exposure to a hazard and the eventual manifestation of disease.

One approach that can help to counter this problem is to carry out the follow up retrospectively. In developing ideas about the fetal origins of coronary heart disease, it was possible to find groups of men and women born in the county of Hertfordshire before 1930 whose fetal and infant growth had been documented. These people were traced, and the cause of death was ascertained for those who had died. Death rates from coronary heart disease could thus be related to weight at birth and at one year old. Obviously, such a study is only feasible when the health outcome of interest can be measured retrospectively. Mortality and cancer incidence can usually be ascertained reliably, but disorders such as asthma may be harder to assess in retrospect. A further requirement is that the selection of exposed people for study should not be influenced by factors related to their subsequent morbidity.

Another modification of the method is to use the recorded disease rates in the national or regional population for control purposes, rather than following up a specially selected control group. This technique is legitimate when exposure to the hazard in the general population is negligible. Thus, in a cohort study of people occupationally exposed to ethylene oxide (used as a sterilant gas and in the manufacture of antifreeze), exposure in the general population was minimal and national death rates could be used as a reference. The numbers of deaths in the cohort were compared with the numbers that would have been expected if subjects had experienced the same death rates specific for age, sex, and calendar period as the general population.

## Clinical follow up studies

What is the prognosis for a 38 year old man who presents with a first epileptic fit, and what advice should he be given about driving? What is the outlook for a manual labourer who has been off work for three months with low back pain? How likely is it that he will be fit to return to his job, and how soon? Questions such as these are investigated by clinical follow up studies—longitudinal studies in which patients with a disease are monitored systematically to establish how their illness progresses and what influences the prognosis.

The need for systematic follow up arises because clinical impressions are often misleading. For example, a neurologist's view of multiple sclerosis tends to be unduly gloomy. Patients in whom the disease remits without residual disability (a third) do not continue to attend that clinic. Those in whom the disease runs a less favourable course return again and again. A general practitioner might be expected to form a more representative impression, but because the disease is rare he will have only a few patients on his list and will not get a complete picture.

For the findings of a clinical follow up study to be generalised to patients elsewhere, it is important to define precisely how subjects are selected for study. For example, patients presenting with asthma to a respiratory physician are likely to have a different prognosis from those seen in general practice. Interpretation is usually easier if entry to follow up is determined by an event (such as first diagnosis) rather than a state (for example, all patients from a renal unit who are on the waiting list for transplants) as outlook for the latter will often vary according to how long they have been in that state. Most studies also document characteristics of subjects when they enter follow up (such as age, sex, and duration and severity of symptoms) so that the influence of these variables on prognosis can be examined.

The methods of follow up are similar to those used in other longitudinal studies and can be prospective or retrospective. For diseases that are often lethal, the outcome may be expressed as case fatality or survival rates. *Case fatality rate* (the proportion of episodes of illness that end fatally) describes the short term outcome of a disease, but must be interpreted with caution. An episode of illness does not correspond to a fixed time interval. Often it refers to a period of medical care, as in a coronary care unit, and case fatality rates may therefore be altered merely by varying the length of stay in hospital. To measure outcome over longer periods, *survival rates* are used. These show the proportion of patients surviving for a specified time from the date of diagnosis or start of treatment. Survival rates may be corrected to allow for deaths from causes other than the disease being studied. By

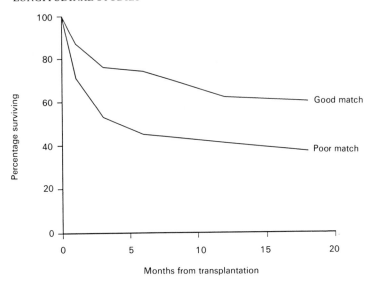

*Survival of kidney grafts according to matching for HLA tissue types*

plotting survival rates at different times it is possible to construct *survival curves*. An example is shown in the figure.

# 8: Case-control and cross sectional studies

## Case-control studies

As discussed in the previous chapter, one of the drawbacks of using a longitudinal approach to investigate the causes of disease with low incidence is that large and lengthy studies may be required to give adequate statistical power. An alternative which avoids this difficulty is the case-control or *case-referent* design. In a case-control study patients who have developed a disease are identified and their past exposure to suspected aetiological factors is compared with that of controls or referents who do not have the disease. This permits estimation of odds ratios (but not of attributable risks). Allowance is made for potential confounding factors by measuring them and making appropriate adjustments in the analysis. This statistical adjustment may be rendered more efficient by matching cases and controls for exposure to confounders, either on an individual basis (for example by pairing each case with a control of the same age and sex) or in groups (for example, choosing a control group with an overall age and sex distribution similar to that of the cases). Unlike in a cohort study, however, matching does not on its own eliminate confounding. Statistical adjustment is still required.

### Selection of cases

The starting point of most case-control studies is the identification of cases. This requires a suitable case definition (see chapter 2). In addition, care is needed that bias does not arise from the way in which cases are selected. A study of benign prostatic hypertrophy might be misleading if cases were identified from hospital admissions and admission to hospital was influenced not only by the presence and severity of disease but also by other variables, such as social class. In general it is better to use incident rather than prevalent cases. As pointed out in chapter 2, prevalence is influenced not only by the risk of developing disease but also by factors that determine the duration of illness. Furthermore, if disease has been present for a long time then premorbid exposure to risk factors may be harder to ascertain, especially if assessment depends on people's memories.

*Selection of controls*

Usually it is not too difficult to obtain a suitable source of cases, but selecting controls tends to be more problematic. Ideally, controls would satisfy two requirements. Within the constraints of any matching criteria, their exposure to risk factors and confounders should be representative of that in the population "at risk" of becoming cases—that is, people who do not have the disease under investigation, but who would be included in the study as cases if they had. Also, the exposures of controls should be measurable with similar accuracy to those of the cases. Often it proves impossible to satisfy both of these aims.

Two sources of controls are commonly used. Controls selected from the general population (for example, from general practice age-sex registers) have the advantage that their exposures are likely to be representative of those at risk of becoming cases. However, assessment of their exposure may not be comparable with that of cases, especially if the assessment is achieved by personal recall. Cases are keen to find out what caused their illness and are therefore better motivated to remember details of their past than controls with no special interest in the study question.

Measurement of exposure can be made more comparable by using patients with other diseases as controls, especially if subjects are not told the exact focus of the investigation. However, their exposures may be unrepresentative. To give an extreme example, a case-control study of bladder cancer and smoking could give quite erroneous findings if controls were taken from the chest clinic. If other patients are to be used as referents, it is safer to adopt a range of control diagnoses rather than a single disease group. In that way, if one of the control diseases happens to be related to a risk factor under study, the resultant bias is not too large.

Sometimes interpretation is helped by having two sets of controls with different possible sources of bias. For example, a link has been suggested between the phenoxy herbicides 2,4-D and 2,4,5-T and soft tissue sarcoma. Some case-control studies to test this have taken referents from the general population, whereas others have used patients with other types of cancer. Studies using controls from the general population will tend to overestimate risk because of differential recall, whereas studies using patients with other types of cancers as controls will underestimate risk if phenoxy herbicides cause cancers other than soft tissue sarcoma. The true risk might therefore be expected to lie somewhere between estimates obtained with the two different designs.

When cases and controls are both freely available then selecting equal numbers will make a study most efficient. However, the number of cases that can be studied is often limited by the rarity of the disease under investigation. In this circumstance statistical confidence can be increased by taking more than one control per case. There is, however, a law of diminishing returns, and it is usually not worth going beyond a ratio of four or five controls to one case.

## Ascertainment of exposure

Many case-control studies ascertain exposure from personal recall, using either a self administered questionnaire or an interview. The validity of such information will depend in part on the subject matter. People may be able to remember quite well where they lived in the past or what jobs they did. On the other hand, long term recall of dietary habits is probably less reliable.

Sometimes exposure can be established from historical records. For example, in a study of the relation between sinusitis and subsequent risk of multiple sclerosis the medical histories of cases and controls were ascertained by searching their general practice notes. Provided that records are reasonably complete, this method will usually be more accurate than one that depends on memory.

Occasionally, long term biological markers of exposure can be exploited. In an African study to evaluate the efficiency of BCG immunisation in preventing tuberculosis, history of inoculation was established by looking for a residual scar on the upper arm. Biological markers are only useful, however, when they are not altered by the subsequent disease process. For example, serum cholesterol concentrations measured after a myocardial infarct may not accurately reflect levels before the onset of infarction.

*Analysis*

The statistical techniques for analysing case-control studies are too complex to cover in a book of this length. Readers who wish to know more should consult more advanced texts or seek advice from a medical statistician.

## Cross sectional studies

A cross sectional study measures the prevalence of health outcomes or determinants of health, or both, in a population at a point in time or over a short period. Such information can be used to explore aetiology—for example, the relation between cataract and vitamin status has been examined in cross sectional surveys. However, associations must be interpreted with caution. Bias may arise because of selection into or out of the study population. A cross sectional survey of asthma in an occupational group of animal handlers would underestimate risk if the development of respiratory symptoms led people to seek alternative employment and therefore to be excluded from the study. A cross sectional design may also make it difficult to establish what is cause and what is effect. If milk drinking is associated with peptic ulcer, is that because milk causes the disease, or because ulcer sufferers drink milk to relieve their symptoms? Because of these difficulties, cross sectional studies of aetiology are best suited to diseases that produce little disability and to the presymptomatic phases of more serious disorders.

Other applications of cross sectional surveys lie in planning health care. For example, an occupational physician planning a coronary prevention programme might wish to know the prevalence of different risk factors in the workforce under his care so that he could tailor his intervention accordingly.

# 9: Experimental studies

The survey designs described in chapters 6 to 8 are all observational. Investigators study people as they find them. Thus, subjects exposed to a risk factor often differ from those who are unexposed in other ways, which independently influence their risk of disease. If such confounding influences are identified in advance then allowing for them in the design and analysis of the study may be possible. There is still, however, a chance of unrecognised confounders.

Experimental studies are less susceptible to confounding because the investigator determines who is exposed and who is unexposed. In particular, if exposure is allocated randomly and the number of groups or individuals randomised is large then even unrecognised confounding effects become statistically unlikely.

There are, of course, ethical constraints on experimental research in humans, and it is not acceptable to expose subjects deliberately to potentially serious hazards. This limits the application of experimental methods in the investigation of disease aetiology, although it may be possible to evaluate preventive strategies experimentally. For example, factories participating in a coronary heart disease prevention project were assigned to two groups, one receiving a programme of screening for coronary risk factors and health education, and the other being left alone. Subsequent disease incidence was then compared between the two groups. The main application of experimental studies, however, is in evaluating therapeutic interventions by randomised controlled trials.

## Randomised controlled trials

At the outset of a randomised controlled trial the criteria for entry to the study sample must be specified (for example, in terms of age, sex, diagnosis, etc). As in other epidemiological investigations, the subjects studied should be representative of the target population in whom it is hoped to apply the results. Comparison of two treatments for rheumatoid arthritis in a series of hospital patients may not provide a reliable guide to managing the less severe range of the disease seen in general practice. Subjects who satisfy the entry criteria are asked to consent to participation. When refusal rates are high a judgement must be made as to how far the volunteers that remain can be considered representative of the target population. They might, for example, be younger on average than the refusers. Is this important in relation to the study question?

Those subjects who agree to participate are then randomised to the treatments under comparison. This can be achieved using published tables of random numbers, or with random numbers generated by computer. When subjects enter the study sequentially (for instance, as they are admitted to hospital) then randomisation is often carried out in blocks. Thus in a study comparing two treatments, A and B, patients might be randomised in blocks of six. Of the first six patients entering the trial, three would be allocated to treatment A and three to treatment B—which patient received which treatment being determined randomly. A similar technique would be used to allocate treatments in each successive set of six patients. The advantage of this method is that it prevents large imbalances in the numbers of patients assigned to different treatments, which otherwise could occasionally occur by chance. It also ensures that the balance between the different treatments is roughly constant throughout the course of the study, thus reducing the opportunity for confounding by extraneous variables that change over time.

Sometimes major determinants of outcome can be identified at the time when subjects enter the study. For example, in a trial of treatment for acute myocardial infarction the presence of certain dysrythmias on admission to hospital might be an important index of prognosis. The use of randomisation means that such prognostic markers will tend to be evenly distributed between the different treatment groups. However, as further insurance against inadvertent confounding, there is the option to stratify subjects at entry according to the prognostic variable (for example, separating patients with and without dysrythmias) and then randomise separately within each stratum in blocks.

When outcome is influenced by other aspects of a patient's management, as well as by the treatments under comparison, it may be desirable for those responsible for management to be "blinded" to which treatment has been allocated. Arrangements must be made, however, to permit rapid unblinding should possible complications of treatment develop. As far as possible, the criteria for withdrawing a patient from treatment should be specified in advance, although final responsibility must rest with the clinical team caring for the patient. Even if a patient is withdrawn from a treatment under investigation, follow up and assessment of outcome should continue.

The end points of trials vary from objective outcomes, such as haemoglobin concentration or birth weight, to more subjective symptoms and physical signs. Bias in the evaluation of subjective outcomes can be avoided by blinding the assessor to the treatment given. For example, if a new analgesic for migraine is being evaluated on the basis of reported levels of symptoms, it may help to use a pharmacologically inactive placebo for comparison. Otherwise, there is a danger that patients will perceive a benefit simply because they are getting something new. Similarly, if the end point is a subjective physical sign (such as severity of a skin rash) then the examiner is best kept ignorant about which patient received which treatment. It is important to measure not only the outcomes that the treatments are intended to improve, but also possible adverse effects. In a trial of the cholesterol lowering drug, clofibrate, the treated group showed a reduced incidence of non-fatal myocardial infarction, but their overall mortality was more than in untreated controls. This excess mortality could not be attributed to any single cause of death, but may have reflected unsuspected side effects of treatment.

The statistical analysis of randomised controlled trials is too complex to cover in a book of this length, and readers who wish to learn about the methods used should consult a more advanced text. Whatever analytical technique is adopted, it is important always to compare subjects according to the treatment to which they were randomised, even if this treatment was not completed. (In some cases it may not even have been started.) Otherwise, the effects of selective withdrawal from treatment may be overlooked. For example, in a trial to compare a β blocker with placebo in an attempt to reduce mortality after myocardial infarction, patients were withdrawn from treatment if they developed severe heart failure – a potential complication of β blockers. The patients most likely to be precipitated into heart failure by the trial drug were those with more severe infarcts and therefore a worse prognosis. Fewer of such patients would be expected to develop heart failure while taking placebo. Thus if the withdrawals had been excluded from the analysis any benefits from the β blocker would have tended to be spuriously exaggerated.

At the same time, it is also helpful to examine outcomes according to treatments actually received. One would be suspicious if the benefits from randomisation to a treatment were confined to those who did not go through with it!

The size of a randomised controlled trial may be decided in advance on the basis of calculated statistical power. Such calculations require specification of the expected distribution of outcome measures, and of the difference in outcomes between treatments that is worth detecting, and are best carried out in collaboration with a medical statistician. A problem with this approach, however, is that the trial may continue long after sufficient data have been accumulated to show that one treatment is clearly superior. Thus some patients would be exposed unnecessarily to suboptimal treatment. A way of avoiding this difficulty is to monitor the results of the trial at intervals, with preset criteria for calling a halt if one treatment appears to be clearly better.

Another problem with randomised controlled trials lies in the need to obtain properly informed consent from participants. Some patients find it hard to understand why a doctor should allocate treatment at random rather than according to his best judgement. This difficulty has prompted an alternative design, which may be applicable when comparing a new treatment with conventional management. Randomisation is carried out for all patients who satisfy the entry criteria, and those who are allocated to conventional treatment are treated in the standard manner. Those assigned to the new treatment are asked to consent to this, but if they refuse are treated conventionally. The need to explain randomisation is thus avoided. Against this, however, must be set two weaknesses. Firstly, as in any randomised experiment, the prime analysis is according to randomisation. If a substantial proportion of patients refuse the new treatment, then differences in outcome may be obscured. Secondly, neither the clinical team nor the patient can be made blind to the treatment received. The importance of this limitation will depend on the nature of the study and the end points being measured.

## Crossover studies

Another modification of the randomised controlled trial is the crossover design. This is particularly useful when outcome is measured by reports of subjective symptoms, but it can only be applied when the effects of treatment are short lived (for example, pain relief from an analgesic).

In a crossover study, eligible patients who have consented to participate receive each treatment sequentially, often with a "wash out" period between treatments to eliminate any carry over effects. However, the order in which treatments are given is randomised so that different patients receive them in different sequence. Outcome is monitored during each period of treatment, and in this way each patient can serve as his own control.

## Experimental study of populations

Most experimental studies allocate and compare treatments between individual subjects, but it is also possible to carry out experimental interventions at the level of populations. We have already cited a coronary heart disease prevention project in which the units of study were the workforces of different factories.

As in studies of individuals, interventions in populations can be randomly allocated. However, if the number of populations under comparison is small then randomisation may not be of much value. Instead, it may be better to assign interventions in a deliberately planned way to ensure maximum comparability between different intervention groups. Control of residual confounding can be strengthened by comparing study and control populations before and after the intervention is introduced.

Like longitudinal studies, experimental investigations tend to be time consuming and expensive. They should not, therefore, be undertaken without good reason. However, if well designed and conducted, they do provide the most compelling evidence of cause and effect.

# 10: Screening

Screening patients for preclinical disease is an established part of day to day medical practice. Routine recording of blood pressure, urine testing, and preoperative chest radiography may all be regarded as screening activities. Increasingly, screening is now being extended to people who have not themselves requested medical aid. For example, general practitioners invite patients who would not otherwise be attending the surgery to undergo tests such as cholesterol measurement and cervical cytology. This places the doctor in a different role, and there is a special obligation to ensure that such screening is beneficial. To this end three questions must be answered, for which epidemiological data are required.

## Does earlier treatment improve the prognosis?

Lung cancers detected at an early stage in their development are more likely to be surgically resectable. Moreover, it is possible to identify such tumours when they are still asymptomatic by chest radiography and sputum cytology. However, a large study in the United States failed to demonstrate any clear reduction in mortality from lung cancer among heavy smokers who were offered four-monthly screening by radiography and sputum cytology, despite the fact that more resectable tumours were detected in the screened population. As this example shows, the outcome of screening must be judged in terms of its effect on mortality or illness, and not simply by the number and severity of cases identified.

Assessing the benefits of early treatment is not always easy. One potential source of error is the phenomenon known as *lead time*.

Suppose that we wish to explore the scope for reducing mortality from breast cancer by early diagnosis. One approach might be to compare the survival of patients whose tumours were detected at screening with that of women who only present once their disease has become symptomatic. However, this could be misleading. Survival might be longer in the screened women not because early treatment is beneficial, but simply because their tumours are being diagnosed earlier in the natural history of their disease (fig).

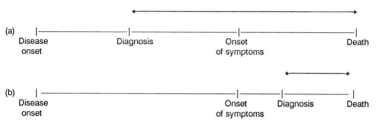

*Lead time (With screening (a) disease is diagnosed earlier than without screening (b) and survival is longer from diagnosis, but this does not necessarily imply that the time course of the disease has been modified.)*

A further difficulty in comparisons of survival is that, apart from any effects of treatment, cases detected at screening tend to be more slowly progressive. Patients with aggressive disease are more likely to develop symptoms in the intervals between screening examinations and therefore present spontaneously.

Outcome is best assessed by systematically comparing the morbidity and mortality of a screened population with that of controls. Moreover, because people who attend for screening may have a different incidence of disease from those who do not, it is important to measure outcome in all of the population selected for screening and not only in those members who actually undergo investigation. Women from social classes IV and V have the highest rates of cervical cancer but the lowest uptake of cervical cytology. Thus an analysis restricted to women undergoing cervical screening would tend to indicate lower mortality even if in fact there was no advantage in early treatment.

## Is a satisfactory screening test available?

Even if prognosis is improved by early treatment, screening is only worthwhile if a satisfactory diagnostic test is available. The test must detect cases in sufficient numbers and at acceptable cost, and it must not carry side effects that outweigh the benefits of screening. Because a screening test must be inexpensive and easy to perform, it is not usually the most valid diagnostic method for a disease. In screening, therefore, it has to be accepted that some cases will remain undetected. As with all diagnostic tests, there is a trade off between sensitivity and specificity, and the competing needs for each must be balanced.

In addition to its sensitivity and specificity, the performance of a test is measured by its *predictive value*. The predictive value of a positive result is the probability that a person who reacts positively to the test actually has the disease. Predictive value varies with the prevalence of disease in the population to whom the test is applied. If the prevalence is low then there are more false positive results than true positives, and predictive value falls. At the extreme, if nobody has the disease then the predictive value will be zero—all positive test results will be false positives. It follows that a test that functions well in normal clinical practice will not necessarily be useful for screening purposes. Sputum cytology has quite a high positive predictive value for bronchial carcinoma in patients presenting with haemoptysis, but if it is used to screen asymptomatic people most positive results will be false.

Because the average benefit to the individual from a screening programme is usually much smaller than from interventions in response to symptoms, screening tests need to be safer than those used in normal clinical practice. The radiation dose from a chest *x* ray examination is small, but if the investigation forms part of a screening programme for tuberculosis, then even the very small risk of complications may outweigh the benefits of early diagnosis. As the prevalence of pulmonary tuberculosis in the general population has declined, so mass radiographic screening has ceased to be justifiable.

## What are the yields of the screening service?

The yield of a screening service is measured by the number of cases identified whose prognosis is improved as a result of their early detection. This must be related to the total number of tests performed. Theoretically, the yields of screening may be improved by restricting it to high risk groups, as has been suggested in the screening of infants for developmental and other abnormalities. But identifying relatively small high risk groups among whom most cases will be found is rarely feasible. If uptake of a screening procedure is low then yield will be correspondingly limited.

Ultimately the yields of a screening service have to be balanced against the costs, in terms of staff and facilities, of screening and making the confirmatory diagnoses. For breast cancer screening it has been found that identifying one case requires examining 170 women by palpation and mammography and taking nine biopsy specimens.

# 11: Outbreaks of disease

Although communicable diseases have declined in industrialised societies, outbreaks of disease such as influenza, gastroenteritis, and hepatitis are still important. During the 1957–8 influenza epidemic, for example, the death rate in England and Wales was 1 per 1000 population above the seasonal average; an estimated 12 million people developed the disease; and the workload of general practitioners increased fivefold. From time to time new communicable diseases such as Lassa fever, legionnaires' disease, and, most recently, AIDS appear in epidemic form.

## Communicable disease outbreaks

In outbreaks of common communicable diseases such as gastroenteritis and hepatitis appropriate investigations must be initiated. The routine for these investigations is also the model for studying non-infectious disease epidemics.

At the outset it is necessary to *verify the diagnosis*. Three patients with halothane induced hepatitis were referred to one university hospital. Investigation of an outbreak of infectious hepatitis was begun, presumably because the clustering of cases gave an impression of infectivity and unduly influenced the physician's diagnosis. With some diseases—Lassa fever, for example—urgency demands that immediate action is taken on the basis of a clinical diagnosis alone. But for most diseases there is less urgency and the doctor should remember that clusters of cases of uncommon non-infectious diseases sometimes occur in one place within a short time simply by chance.

From time to time errors in collecting, handling, or processing laboratory specimens may cause "pseudo epidemics". The Centers for Disease Control in Atlanta, Georgia, USA, have reported several such pseudo epidemics. In one, an apparent outbreak of typhoid occurred when specimen contamination produced blood cultures positive for *Salmonella typhi* in six patients.

If a disease is endemic (habitually present in a community) it is necessary to estimate its previous frequency and thereby *confirm an increase in incidence* above the normal endemic level. Pseudo epidemics may arise from sudden increases in doctors' or patients' awareness of a disease, or from changes in the organisation of a doctor's practice. When the endemic level has been defined from incidences over previous weeks, months, or years the rate of increase of incidence above this level may indicate whether the epidemic is contagious or has arisen from a point source. Contagious epidemics emerge gradually whereas point source epidemics, such as occur when many people are exposed more or less simultaneously to a source of pathogenic organisms, arise abruptly.

To build up a description of an epidemic it will be necessary to take case histories to identify the *characteristics of the patients*. Patients whose diseases are notified or otherwise recorded are often only a proportion of those with the disease, and additional cases must be sought. Thereafter it is necessary to *define the population at risk*, and relate the cases to this. This will require mapping of the geographical extent of the epidemic.

Defining the population at risk enables the extent and severity of the epidemic to be expressed in terms of attack rates—which may be given either as crude rates, relating the numbers of cases to the total population, or as age and sex specific rates. It may be possible to identify an experience that is common to people affected by the disease but not shared by those not affected; and, from this, a hypothesis about the source and spread of the epidemic may be formulated.

## Modern epidemics

There are several examples of large scale epidemics due to chemical contaminants. Outbreaks of mercury poisoning, with resulting deaths and permanent neurological disability, have been reported from non-industrial countries as a result of ingestion of flour and wheat seed treated with methyl and ethyl mercury compounds. In 1981 in Spain 20 000 people were affected by a new disease, named the "toxic allergic syndrome", the most striking feature of which was a pneumonitis. During the first four months of the epidemic more than 100 people died and 13 000 were treated in hospital. Epidemiological and clinical investigation showed that the cause was ingestion of olive oil adulterated with contaminated rape seed oil.

Widespread environmental contamination is a new agent of epidemic disease. During the 1980s, 26 epidemics of hospital admission for asthma occurred in the city of Barcelona. Epidemiological investigations eventually established that the cause was allergy to soya bean dust released into the atmosphere when cargoes of beans were unloaded in the harbour.

Increasing recognition of environmental hazards from substances introduced by man into his environment, as a result of the application of new technology, has led to a demand for large scale monitoring systems based on automated record linkage. Whether or not such systems come into operation, clinicians' awareness of changes in disease frequency or of the appearance of clusters of unusual cases will continue to be crucial to the early detection of new epidemics. Clinicians have a special responsibility in the early detection of epidemics caused by medication. The rise in mortality during the 1960s among asthmatic patients who used pressurised aerosols, and the occurrence of corneal damage, rashes, and various other adverse effects of practolol are two of many examples of epidemics resulting from prescription of new drugs.

## New diseases

New diseases continue to appear. The name legionnaires' disease was given to an outbreak of pneumonia at a convention of American Legionnaires in Philadelphia, Pennsylvania, USA, in 1976. There were 29 deaths. This stimulated an intensive epidemiological investigation whose successful outcome was the identification of a Gram negative bacillus as the causative agent.

From 1981 to 1983 some 2000 cases of AIDS were reported in the USA. The ratio of men to women was 15 to 1, and the epidemiology suggested an infectious agent usually transmitted by homosexual intercourse. AIDS seemed to be a new disease. Subsequent studies, however, showed it to be endemic in central Africa but with a sex ratio of around 1 to 1, which suggested spread by heterosexual contact. Investigations of this kind are a dramatic application of epidemiology.

# 12: Reading epidemiological reports

Epidemiological methods are widely applied in medical research, and even doctors who do not themselves carry out surveys will find that their clinical practice is influenced by epidemiological observations. Which oral contraceptive is the best option for a woman of 35? What prognosis should be given to parents whose daughter has developed spinal scoliosis? What advice should be given to the patient who is concerned about newspaper reports that living near electric power lines causes cancer? To answer questions such as these, the doctor must be able to understand and interpret epidemiological reports.

Interpretation is not always easy, and studies may produce apparently inconsistent results. One week a survey is published suggesting that low levels of alcohol intake reduce mortality. The next, a report concludes that any alcohol at all is harmful. How can such discrepancies be reconciled? This chapter sets out a framework for the assessment of epidemiological data, breaking the exercise down into three major components.

## Bias

The first step in evaluating a study is to identify any major potential for bias. Almost all epidemiological studies are subject to bias of one sort or another. This does not mean that they are scientifically unacceptable and should be disregarded. However, it is important to assess the probable impact of biases and to allow for them when drawing conclusions. In what direction is each bias likely to have affected outcome, and by how much?

If the study has been reported well, the investigators themselves will have addressed this question. They may even have collected data to help quantify bias. In a survey of myopia and its relation to reading in childhood, information was gathered about the use of spectacles and the educational history of subjects who were unavailable for examination. This helped to establish the scope for bias from the incomplete response. Usually, however, evaluation of bias is a matter of judgement.

When looking for possible biases, three aspects of a study are particularly worth considering:

(1) How were subjects selected for investigation, and how representative were they of the target population with regard to the study question?

(2) What was the response rate, and might responders and non-responders have differed in important ways? As with the choice of the study sample, it matters only if respondents are atypical in relation to the study question.

(3) How accurately were exposure and outcome variables measured? Here the scope for bias will depend on the study question and on the pattern of measurement error. Random errors in assessing intelligence quotient (IQ) will produce no bias at all if the aim is simply to estimate the mean score for a population. On the other hand, in a study of the association between low IQ and environmental exposure to lead, random measurement errors would tend to obscure any relation—that is, to bias estimates of relative risk towards one. If the errors in measurement were non-random, the bias would be different again. For example, if IQs were selectively under-recorded in subjects with high lead exposure, the effect would be to exaggerate risk estimates.

There is no simple formula for assessing biases. Each must be considered on its own merits in the context of the study question.

## Chance

Even after biases have been taken into account, study samples may be unrepresentative just by chance. An indication of the potential for such chance effects is provided by statistical analysis.

Traditionally, statistical inference has been based on hypothesis testing. This can most easily be understood if the study sample is viewed in the context of the larger target population about which conclusions are to be drawn. A *null hypothesis* about the target population is formulated. Then starting with this null hypothesis, and with the assumption that the study sample is an unbiased subset of the target population, a p value is calculated. This is the probability of obtaining an outcome in the study sample as extreme from the null hypothesis as that observed, simply by chance. For example, in a case-control study of the relation between renal stones and dietary oxalate, the null hypothesis might be that in the target population from which the study sample was derived there is no association between renal stones and oxalate intake. A p value of 0·05 would imply that under this assumption of no overall association between renal stones and oxalate, the probability of selecting a random sample in which the association was as strong as that observed in the study would be one in 20. The lower the calculated p value, the more one is inclined to reject the null hypothesis and adopt a contrary view—for example, that there is an association between dietary oxalate and renal stones. Often a p value below a stated threshold (for example, 0·05) is deemed to be (*statistically*) *significant*, but this threshold is arbitrary. There is no reason to attach much greater importance to a p value of 0·049 than to a value of 0·051.

A p value depends not only on the magnitude of any deviation from the null hypothesis, but also on the size of the sample in which that deviation was observed. Failure to achieve a specified level of statistical significance will have different implications according to the size of the study. A common error is to weigh "positive" studies, which find an association to be significant, against "negative" studies, in which it is not. Two case-control studies could indicate similar odds ratios, but because they differed in size one might be significant and the other not. Clearly such findings would not be incompatible.

Because of the limitations of the p value as a summary statistic, epidemiologists today prefer to base statistical inference on confidence intervals. A *statistic* of the study sample, such as an odds ratio or a mean haemoglobin concentration, provides an estimate of the corresponding population *parameter* (the odds ratio or mean haemoglobin concentration in the target population from which the sample was derived). Because the study sample may by chance be atypical, there is uncertainty about the estimate. A confidence interval is a range within which, assuming there are no biases in the study method, the true value for the population parameter might be expected to lie. Most often, *95% confidence intervals* are calculated. The formula for the 95% confidence interval is set in such a way that on average 19 out of 20 such intervals will include the population parameter. Large samples are less prone to chance error than small samples, and therefore give tighter confidence intervals.

Whether statistical inference is based on hypothesis testing or confidence intervals, the results must be viewed in context. Assessment of the contribution of chance to an observation should also take into account the findings of other studies. An epidemiological association might be highly significant statistically, but if it is completely at variance with the balance of evidence from elsewhere, then it could still legitimately be attributed to chance. For example, if a cohort study with no obvious biases suggested that smoking protected against lung cancer, and no special explanation could be found, we would probably conclude that this was a fluke result. Unlike p values or confidence intervals, the weight that is attached to evidence from other studies cannot be precisely quantified.

## Confounding versus causality

If an association is real and not explained by bias or chance, the question remains as to how far it is causal and how far the result of confounding. The influence of some confounders may have been eliminated by matching or by appropriate statistical analysis. However, especially in observational studies, the possibility of unrecognised residual confounding remains. Assessment of whether an observed association is causal depends in part on what is known about the biology of the relation. In addition, certain characteristics of the association may encourage a causal interpretation. A dose-response relation in which risk increases progressively with higher exposure is generally held to favour causality, although in theory it might arise through confounding. In the case of hazards suspected of acting early in a disease process, such as genotoxic carcinogens, a latent interval between first exposure and the manifestation of increased risk would also support a causal association. Also important is the magnitude of the association as measured by the relative risk or odds ratio. If an association is to be completely explained by confounding then the confounder must carry an even higher relative risk for the disease and also be strongly associated with the exposure under study. A powerful risk factor with, say, a 10-fold relative risk for the disease would probably be recognised and identified as a potential confounder.

The evaluation of possible pathogenic mechanisms and the importance attached to dose-response relations and evidence of latency are also a matter of judgement. It is because there are so many subjective elements to the interpretation of epidemiological findings that experts do not always agree. However, if sufficient data are available then a reasonable consensus can usually be achieved.

# Further reading

Armitage P, Berry G. *Statistical Methods in Medical Research*. Oxford: Blackwell, 1994. A full and explicit reference work on statistics.

Barker D J P, Hall A J. *Practical Epidemiology*. Edinburgh: Churchill Livingstone, 1991. A short practical manual of epidemiology for use in developing countries.

Coggon D. *Statistics in Clinical Practice*. London: BMJ Publishing Group, 1995. A guide to the interpretation of medical statistics for non-mathematicians.

Gardner M J, Altman D G. *Statistics with Confidence*. London: British Medical Journal, 1989. A clearly written, short introduction to statistical methods.

Pocock S J. *Clinical Trials: a Practical Approach*. Chichester: Wiley, 1996. A detailed guide to clinical trials.

Rothman K J. *Modern Epidemiology*. Boston: Little, Brown, 1986. The most rigorous exposition of epidemiological concepts and principles.

Swinscow T D V. *Statistics at Square One*. London: revised by Campbell M J. BMJ Publishing Group, 1996. Medical statistics made as simple as possible.

# Index